THE GODLY FIT COOKING GUIDE FOR KINGDOM LIVING

THE
GODLY FIT
COOKING GUIDE
FOR
KINGDOM LIVING

TIFFANY BOSTIC

Disclaimer: It is important that you seek appropriate medical advice before starting any regimen or dietary needs discussed in this book. You are responsible for all decisions pertaining to your health. The writer and publisher of this cookbook are not responsible for adverse reactions, effects, or consequences resulting from the use of any recipes or suggestions herein or hereafter. To obtain the most accurate nutritional information in any recipe, please calculate the nutritional information based on the ingredients, and brands that you use in your recipe.

Printed in the United States of America

Cover Designer: Kozakura
Editor: LPW Editing & Consulting Services, LLC
        www.litapward.com

First Printing, 2019

ISBN – 9781798593332

ACKNOWLEDGEMENTS

The completion of this book could not have been possible if it wasn't for my Lord and Savior, who is first in every area of my life.

To my wonderful husband and children, you guys push me every day to be great! I love you and there is nothing I wouldn't do for you.

Thanks to all of my clients for believing in me and allowing me to be a part of your fitness journey.

To my best friend/assistant, thank you for believing in me and pushing me daily to pursue my purpose.

Special thanks to my sisters in Christ, Carol Clark, Phyllis Scarborough and Carol Bruce Gage for being in the right place at the right time to confirm the title of this cookbook. I love you ladies.

Finally, Apostle Shirley R. Brown, and the late Apostle Carolyn James who has poured so much wisdom and spiritually guidance into me, and has confirmed my purpose in the Kingdom. I love you to life.

TABLE OF CONTENTS

INTRODUCTION

This simple, yet informative guide is designed to help individuals become *Godly fit*. Much of the information has been gleamed from experience and teaching that Coach T acquired over a period of 10 years. The information has been strategically organized to help anyone who has a desire to be spiritually, physically and emotionally fit for the Kingdom. *Godly Fit* is a process of detoxing your mind and body from negative energy and impurities that will keep you from complete wholeness. May this simple, quick guide help individuals obtain clarity on becoming fit for the Kingdom.

For physical training is of some value, but godliness has value for all things holding promise for both the present life and the life to come. (1 Timothy 4:8 NIV)

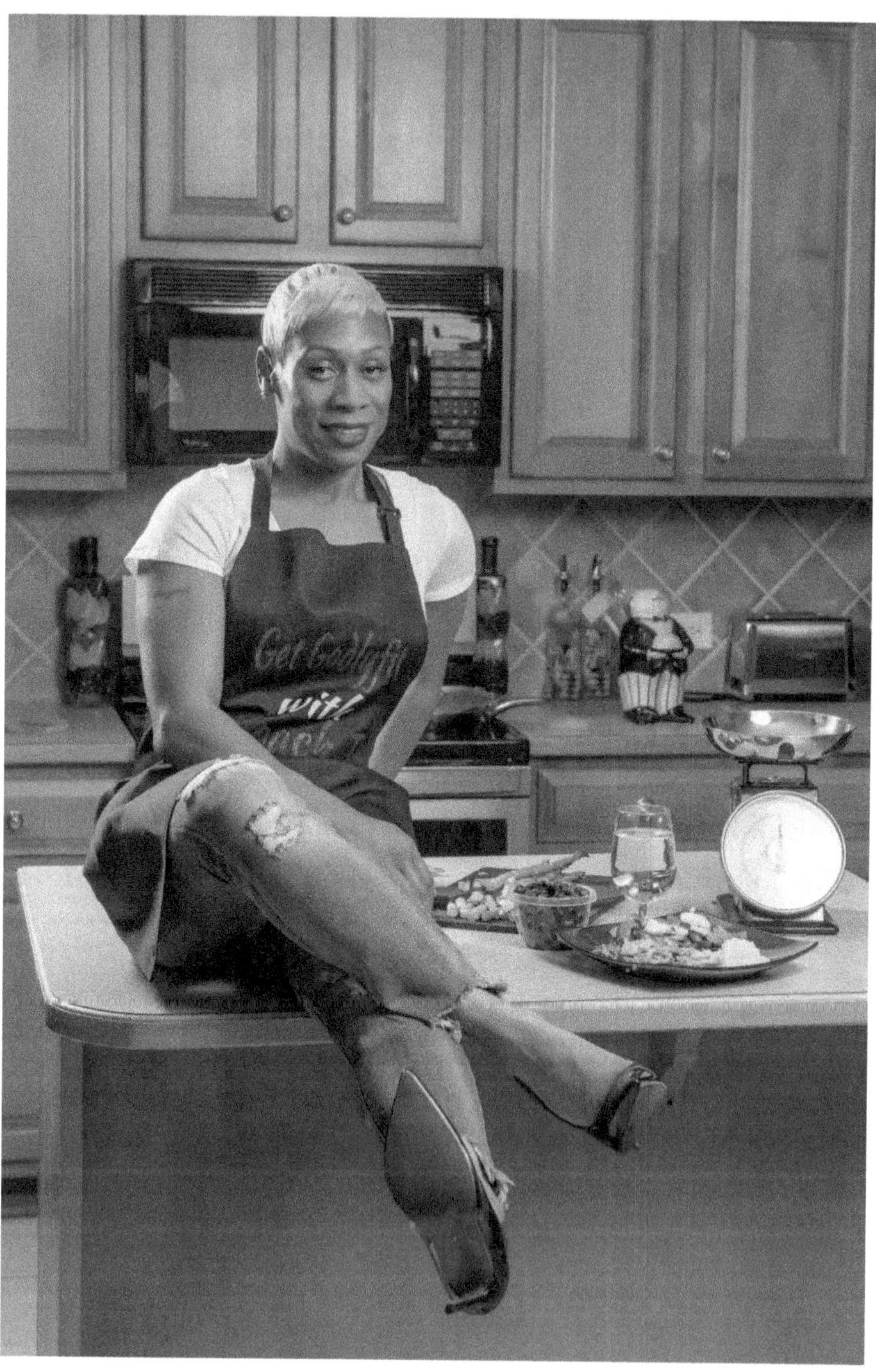

COACH T'S PHILOSPHY ON NUTRITION

Now days, everyone has an opinion on proper nutrition. The most common word I hear when it comes to nutrition is the word diet. There are several extremes like the Paleo diet that will not allow you to eat grains or legumes or diary. Vegan diets will not allow you to eat animal products. The South Beach diet, the Zone diet, the Atkins diet, and the Cabbage Soup diet? What about Weight Watchers, Jenny Craig, Herbal Life, Iaso Tea, and Isogenic? All of the information advertised is confusing. No wonder the nation is the fattest it has been! Most of the time people are trying to figure out which diet to choose, and over time they throw in the towel and go back to their old eating habits.

I've tried several different diet plans myself. I've lost the weight without drinking sodas, counting calories, and the no carb diet. I consider myself experienced with dieting experimentation.

However, there is one philosophy that has made me feel better, look better and have greater results than any other diet that I have ever come across. It's the philosophy that I created, the *Godly Fit* way. It may not be profound, but when you think about it, maybe you haven't seen it this way. Here are some tools to consider when grocery shopping and meal planning.

Eat Whole Foods: Stay on the perimeter of the grocery store. If the item(s) is in a box and there are ingredients you do not recognize, then you should skip it. Choose foods with the least amount of ingredients as possible.

Drink Plenty of Water: Your primary drink should be water throughout the day. Of course, you may enjoy coffee or tea in moderation, but mostly water. Half your body weight is ideal.

Sugar: Stay away from refined sugar. Cakes, pies, soda, cookies, high-fructose corn syrup, cane juice or evaporated juice.

Trans Fat: Mainly found in processed foods which has an infinite shelf life; found in margarines, cookies and candy. It will be listed as partially hydrogenated oil. The body does not recognize it as food and doesn't know how to break it down.

Processed and Added Ingredients Food: If it's in a box or bag, it's considered processed. Some frozen or bagged food may be okay from stores like Fresh Market or Trader Joes, but make sure to read the labels and recognize the ingredients. Avoid artificial sweetener and color/flavors.

Fried Food: Anything fried, stay away from.

What about the foods we tend to stay away from? Here are some foods that can accompany your veggies in small portions.

Grains: Make sure the grains are whole grain; 100% whole wheat, brown rice, etc.

Meat: Omit processed meat such as bologna, hotdogs and red hots. The more lean the meat, the better. Make sure to measure the meats, not to over eat. 3-5 oz. in portion size is standard depending on the goal. Eating fish, lean chicken and unprocessed meats are much healthier.

Dairy: Limit your dairy intake to a small amount per day. Choose Almond or Coconut milk instead of dairy milk. Choose natural creamers for coffee.

Alcohol: Limit yourself to 1-2 drinks per week. If you have to have a drink, choose 1 low carb beer or dry red wine. Bourbon or whiskey is not too bad, however, remember too much alcohol will affect the waist line.

This information does not cover every question concerning nutrition, however, it does provide different examples of healthy eating, grocery shopping and food ingredients.

Each person's body and metabolism is different, choose foods that work for you, and stick to them. Stay away from "diets". Change your mind set and make a life style change instead of using different diets. Think about what you are doing to your body while eating. You are either feeding the disease or fighting against it. This philosophy will work for most people. This has worked well for my clients and myself. I am not a certified nutritionist, however I am sharing with you the steps, guide, and information that I know works. The *Godly fit* way has worked for over 40 of my clients, I challenge you to start today to become *Godly Fit*!

In the bible, the number 7 is one of the most significant numbers, because of its spiritual perfection. I have created 7 steps for you as a guide, when you start your Godly fit journey: Commitment, Detoxing, Daily Devotion, Workouts, Fasting, Studying the Word, and Prayer.

<u>GODLY FIT'S 7 STEPS:</u>

1. Commitment: The quality of being dedicated to a cause or activity. Commit yourself to start a healthier lifestyle by making small adjustments to your diet and repeat for 21 days to form a habit.

2. Detox: To abstain from or rid the body of toxic or unhealthy substance. This includes negative energy, negative talk, impurities or anything that is not edifying to the body of Christ.

3. Daily Devotion: Devote yourself to 15-30 minutes which include you and God. Ask Him to keep your body from impurities and anything that is not of spiritual substance for your temple.

4. Moderate Exercise: At least 150 minutes per week of aerobic activity such as brief walking, swimming, working in the garden or vigorous activity like running or dancing.

5. Fasting: A biblical way to truly humble yourself in the sight of God. Instead of burning off food that you just ate, fasting allows your body to tap into reserves. Once you commit to your sacrifice, stick to what you are dedicated to and be sure to ready your Word, pray, study and meditate.

6. Study: God's Word is fully sufficient to prepare us for everything we need regarding keeping the temple clean. Dedicate one hour per day to show yourself approved.

7. Prayer: A request for help or expression of thanks addressed to God. Set aside time before you start your day to seek Him for whatever your heart desires regarding your journey.

I am convinced that if you include these 7 steps as you become Godly fit, you will be more confident, gain mental strength, be able to identify weaknesses and strengths, develop a strong prayer life and know your purpose in the Kingdom.

14 BASIC WAYS TO STICK TO THE GODLY FIT PLAN

The *Godly Fit Plan* will help you physically, mentally and spiritually. It can also help your moods and reduce or eliminate all prescription medications. Without proper coaching and despite the benefits, maintaining a healthy life style change can be difficult. I have created 14 ways to stick to the *Godly Fit Plan*.

1. Set Realistic Goals: Do not have the mind set to lose weight too quickly. Give yourself a tangible number to lose every 4-6 weeks and work towards that goal. In my years of coaching clients, I found that the higher they set the goal, the more likely they would drop the program after the first month. The more realistic the goal, it's a better chance for greater weight loss.

2. Find A Motivator: It is helpful to find a picture of yourself that can help you stay motivated during your journey. Keep this picture handy to refer to when you need a reminder.

3. Keep The Junk Foods Out: It's hard to stay on track when you are surrounded by junk food. Let family and friends know your goal and ask if they would keep the junk food out of sight. Keeping foods out of sight gives you a higher chance of staying on track.

4. Have A Positive Attitude: Just because you bite a cookie or taste the food at a party does not mean you have ruined your healthy lifestyle. Remember not to over indulge. Choose protein packed choices to make you feel full and satisfied instead of lethargic, sluggish and disappointed.

5. Carry Your Prep Bag: The more prepared you are for the day, the higher your changes of staying on track. Not having your meal prep bag will cause you to grab anything available. Consider having healthy snacks on hand just in case you can't eat a full meal. Examples: Greek yogurt, boiled eggs, veggie sticks and almonds.

6. Switch Up Meal Plans and Exercise: In my experience of being a weight loss/prep coach, diet changes and exercising will coincide with each other to produce better results.

7. Have A Plan Before Eating Out: Trying to stay on track while eating out can be challenging. Always have a plan before you get to the restaurant to stay on track. Here are some examples: Eat a healthy snack before you arrive. Drink water with lemon, order food plain, eat sensible, order a salad, chew slowly, and drink black coffee instead of sweets. No buffets, no bread, split a meal with a friend, stay away from creamy sauces, keep your goals in mind.

8. Don't Let Traveling Hinder You: Traveling for work or pleasure can be difficult when trying to stay on track with healthy eating. A few pointers to keep in mind: Challenge yourself to stay on track and pack foods that won't spoil easily.

9. Practice Mindful Eating: Studies show that overweight and obese women who practice mindful eating had significant improvement with their food in a 4-month period.

10. Track Progress: Keeping track of your progress provides motivation that can help keep you going. Take pictures of your progress every 4 weeks. Often times we don't see our progress because we look at ourselves daily, but pictures don't lie.

11. Get An Accountable Workout Partner: Sticking to your plan can be tough on your own, but having a motivating spouse or partner can be helpful.

12. Never Skip Breakfast: If your first meal is packed with protein, this will help maintain blood sugar levels and will prevent over eating for the rest of the day.

13. Don't Rush Your Process: Don't get discouraged on your weight loss journey. Researchers have found that it takes 66 days, on average to make a new behavior a habit.

14. Stick To What Works Best For You: Everyone's body is different, so what works for one person may not work for another person. Develop your eating habit and stick to it. The best plan is the plan you can continue in the long run.

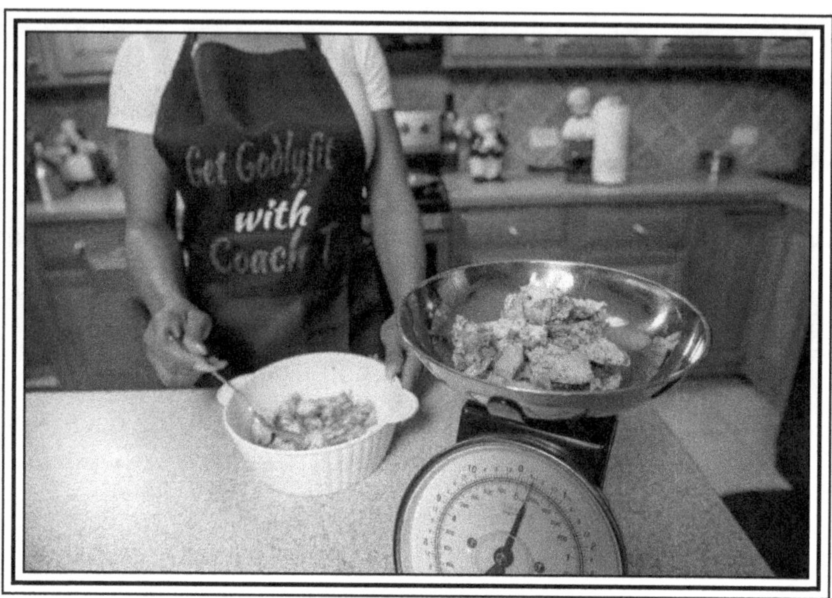

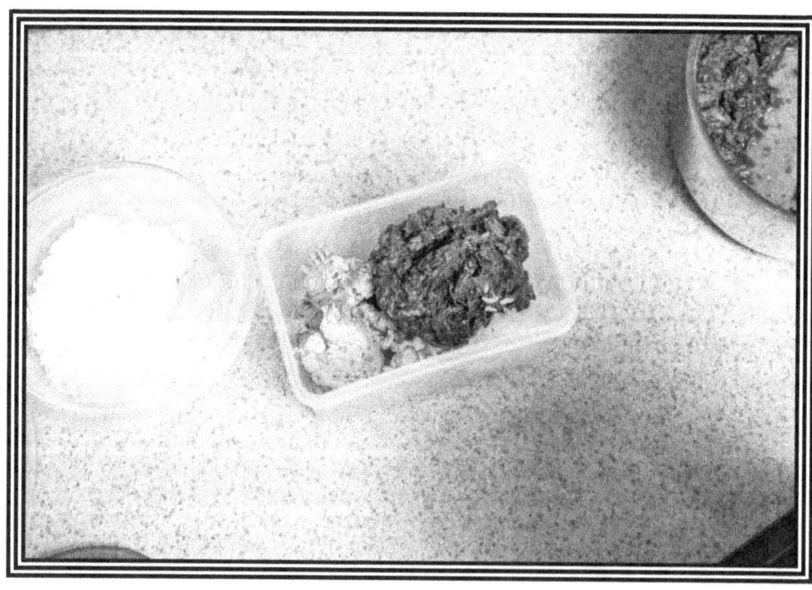

MEAL PREP GUIDE

A Simple Meal Prep Guide: The most important thing to remember is not to get overwhelmed as a beginner. Sticking to the basics will be beneficial. Start by prepping foods you already know. People go on health kicks all the time and soon lose their motivation because they are trying to do too many things in one week. Here are a few tips to help you:

Pick a Day to Prep Meals: As a coach, I give my clients two days per week of rest to prepare their meals. For example, Sundays and Wednesdays. This method will help you stay on track and split meals up too. Keep meals fresh.

Make a List for Your Foods: Decide what meals you're going to prepare for the week and shop for these items only. If you are preparing for a family, choose that you can cook a different meal for them separately. Ex: If you are having fish and asparagus, make your family fish tacos with a low calorie tortilla wrap.

Have Proper Tools and Containers: You can't successfully meal prep without a food scale or containers. You don't want to throw things inside of a big bowl; this defeats the entire purpose of preparing meals. You need containers with sections, which will help with proper portions to prevent over eating. Purchase containers that are "BPA Free" which means safe to use in the microwave. Also, be mindful that same size containers give you the benefit of stacking them easily to have room in the fridge.

Keep It Simple: Focus on simple meals that are easy to prepare. Ex: chicken and fish. Both can be seasoned and prepared in many different ways. Chicken is one of my favorite things to prep because I can freeze it.

Multi-task: You can make so many different things at one time, but try and skip the microwave. Use your oven or you can use a crock pot at the same time. The aluminum pans from the Dollar Tree are great for the oven. Be sure to check your utensils and pans when preparing for your shopping trip.

Seasonings: Eating the same foods sometimes may become boring but different seasonings will help you to stay on track more easily. Seasonings like Mrs. Dash come in different flavors. I recommend purchasing them all. Lemon juice, fresh herbs and spices, red pepper flakes are fine too. Hot sauce, spicy, mustard, and sugar free BBQ sauce are okay in moderation. 1 tablespoon is a perfect amount for those.

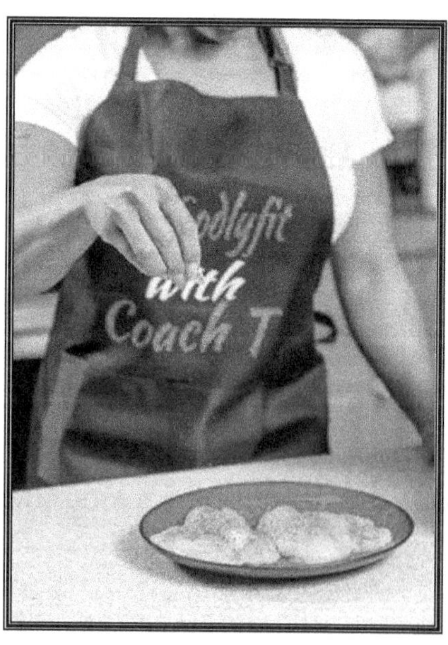

<u>GODLY FIT SMOOTHIES</u>

Arise and Soar
¾ papaya
¾ sliced peaches
½ pear
1 teaspoon Fresh ginger
2 mint Leaves
1 cup of ice (optional)
½ - 1 cup of water to thin
Blend until desired consistency.

Morning Glory
¾ cup blueberries fresh or frozen
¾ cup cherries
½ cup strawberries fresh or frozen
1 tablespoon of flax seed
1 cup of ice (optional)
½ - 1 cup of water to thin
Blend until desired consistency.

Royalty
1/3 cup blueberries fresh or frozen
1/3 cup raspberries fresh or frozen
1/3 cup pomegranate kernels
¼ cup good probiotic juice (optional)
½ banana
½ - 1 cup of water to thin
1 cup of ice (optional)
Blend until desired consistency.

The Revealer
1 banana
1 tablespoon of natural peanut butter or almond butter
1 cup of spinach
½ teaspoon cinnamon
1 cup of cashew or almond milk

½ cup of ice (optional)
Blend until desired consistency.

Victory Detox
1 cup coconut water or regular milk
½ avocado peeled and pitted
1 cup baby spinach
½ green apple
½ cup fresh pineapple chunks
¼ cup celery
1/8 teaspoon ginger
11 tablespoons fresh lemon juice

Spiritual Immune Boost
1 cup unsweet almond or cashew milk
2 large oranges peeled
½ teaspoon vanilla extract
1 tablespoon scoop vanilla low carb protein
1 cup of ice
Blend until desired consistency.

Breakthrough
½ cup kale
½ cup spinach
1 cup coconut water
1 peeled pear
1 peeled apple
½ cup frozen mango chunks
½ cup ice
Blend until desired consistency.

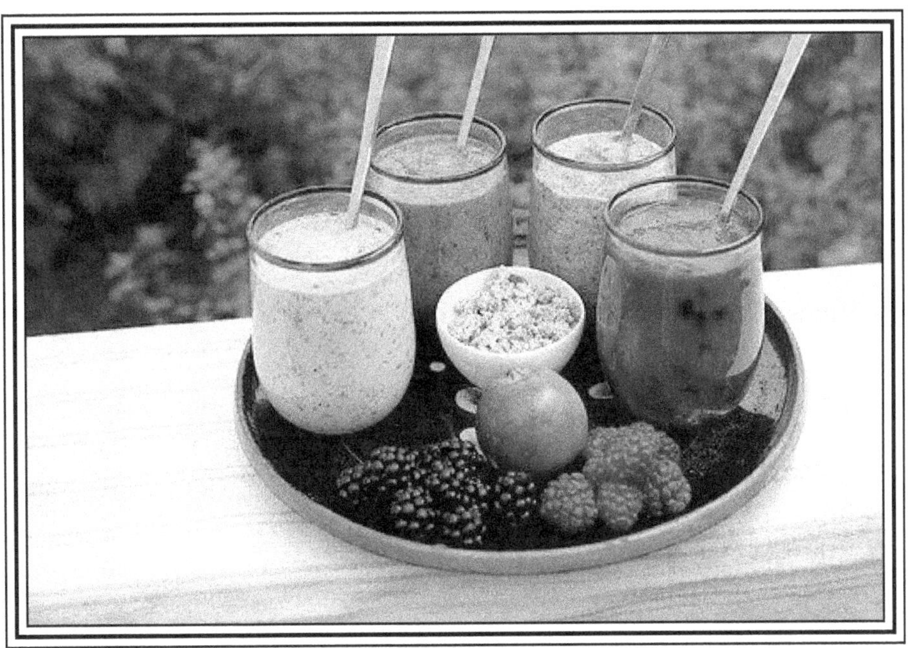

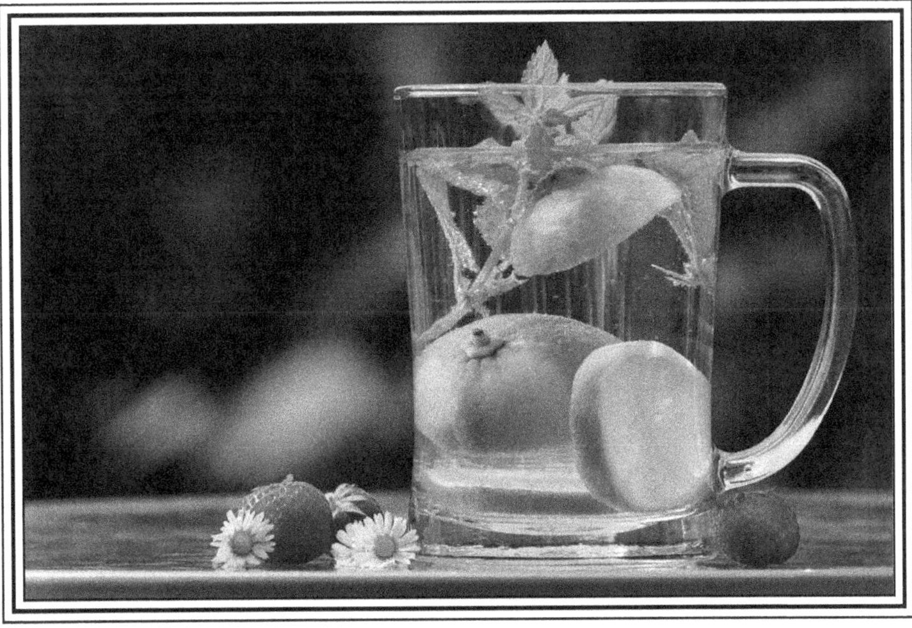

<u>INFUSED WATER RECIPES</u>

Strawberry and Mint
16 strawberries thinly sliced
8 mint sprigs
1-quart water and ice
Chill and serve after 35 minutes

Pineapple and Mint
6 pineapple slices
2 mint sprigs
1-quart water and ice
Serve immediately

Apple Cinnamon Stick
1 large apple chopped
2 cinnamon sticks
1-quart water
Warm 1 cup for 30 seconds in microwave
Or chill and serve

Orange, Cucumber, Lime and Lemon
3 quarts of water
½ orange sliced
½ cucumber sliced
½ lemon sliced
½ lime sliced
Chill and serve.

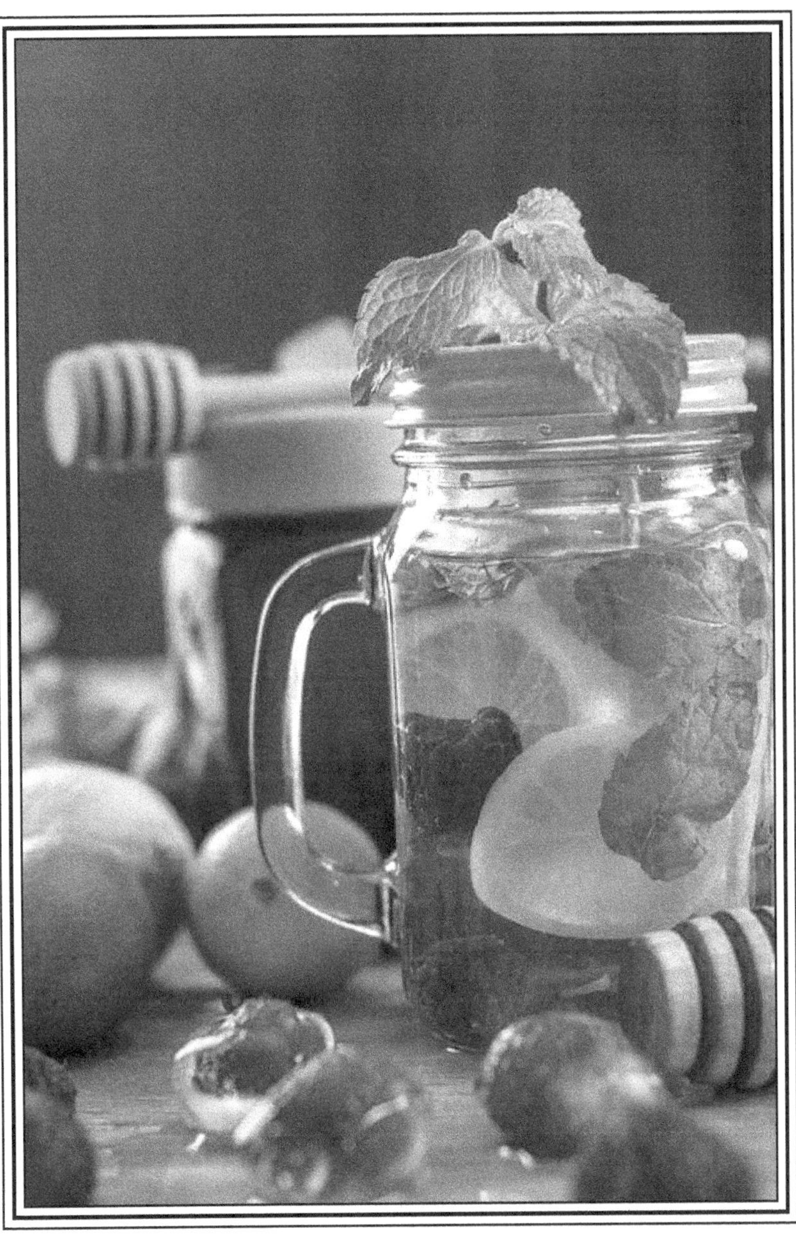

<u>HEALTHY SNACKS</u>

Protein Cinnamon Muffins
1 scoop quest baking protein (cinnamon crunch)
½ cup plain or steel cut oats
3 oz. ripe banana
20 grams sliced almonds
60 grams of egg whites
Unsweetened almond milk for consistency
1 teaspoon of cinnamon

Directions: Bake at 350 degrees. Mix all ingredients after slicing bananas. Spray muffin pan with olive oil or any nonstick spray. Bake for 15 minutes.

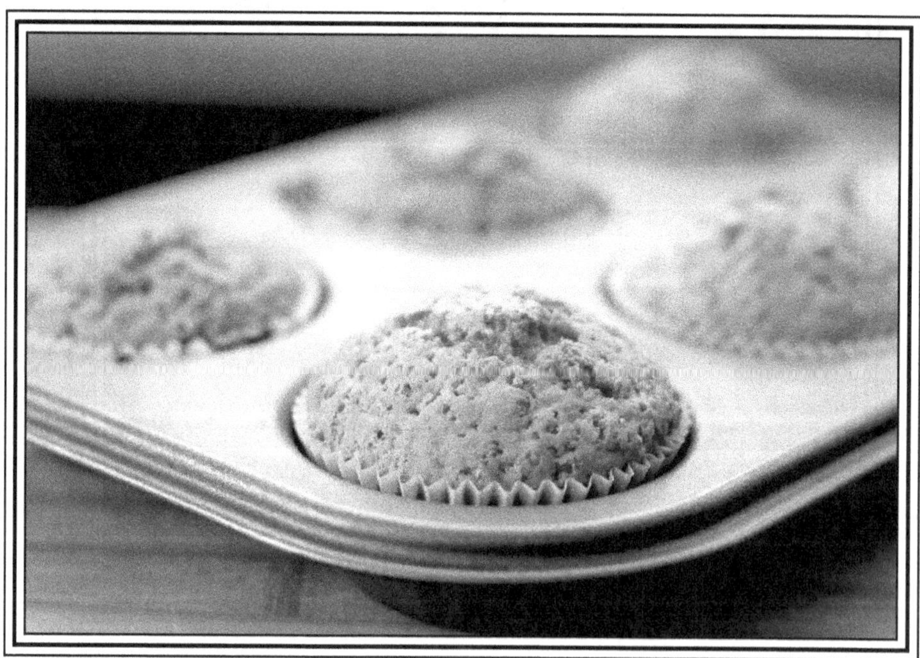

Protein Pancakes
½ scoop quest cinnamon crunch protein
½ cup egg white
1/3 cup oats

Directions: Mix with a spoon and ladle ¼ into a nonstick skillet until bubbles form then flip. Serve with ¼ cup of Walden Farms syrup. You may use 35 grams of your choice of frozen berries, melt in microwave on two 30 second intervals.

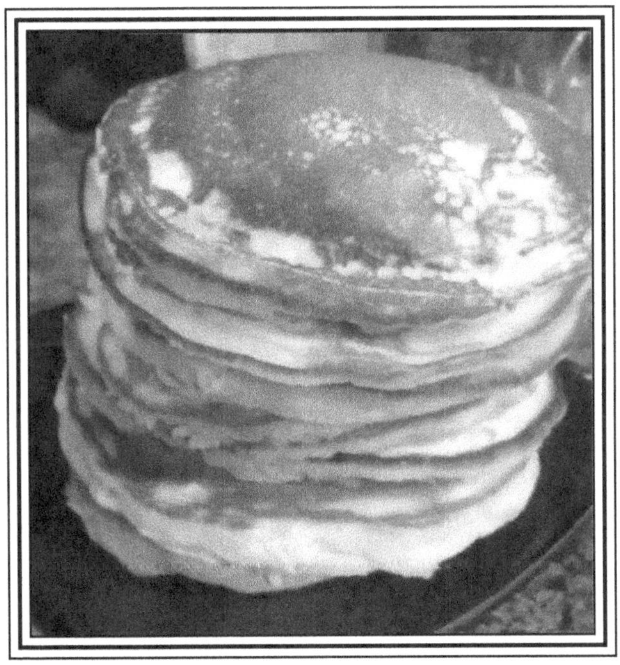

Chocolate Chip/Peanut Butter/Oatmeal Energy Bites
1 cup of natural peanut butter
¼ cup pure maple syrup
2 teaspoons vanilla extract (McCormick)
1 ½ cup quick rolled oats
½ cup unsweetened coconut
1/3 cup organic cacao nibs (Navitas Brand)
2-4 teaspoon of unsweetened almond milk

Directions: Mix peanut butter, maple syrup and vanilla extract. Stir in oats until well combined, add cacao nibs. To create well-formed dough, add 1 teaspoon of almond milk at a time. Use a tablespoon to form more bites. Store in container; they keep for 1 week in fridge and 1 month in freezer.

Chef Notes: I use McCormick and Navitas brand.

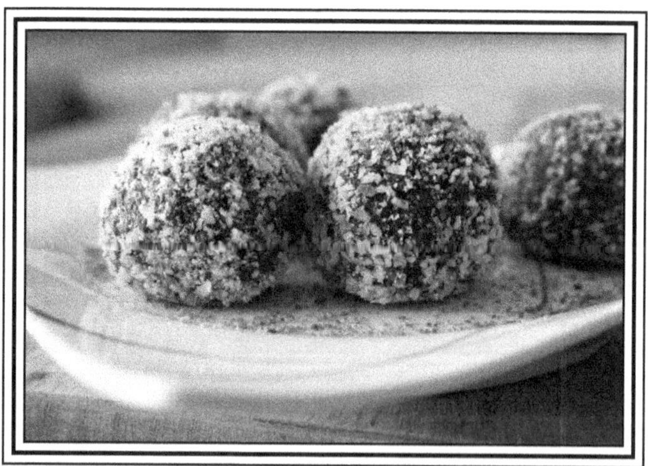

<u>SOUPS</u>

Immune Turmeric Boost
2 tablespoons extra-virgin olive oil
1 ½ cup chopped onion
3 celery stalks
2 large carrots thinly sliced
8 oz. Bella mushrooms
10 garlic cloves minced
8 cups unsalted organic chicken broth
2 Bay leaves
15 oz. can of drained chick peas
2 lbs. chicken breast chopped
1 tablespoon of sea salt
½ teaspoon crushed red pepper (optional)
12 oz. Kale, (remove stems, chopped)

Directions: Heat oil in Dutch oven over medium heat, add onion, carrots, celery until onion turn brown 5 minutes. Add in mushrooms and garlic. Pour in broth, bag leaves, chick peas, simmer. Add dice chicken, salt pepper. Cover for 30 minutes. Remove bay leaves, add kale let simmer for 7 minutes. Enjoy.

Chicken Noodle Soup
1 tablespoon olive oil
2 medium leeks
2 sliced carrots
2 large celery stalks chopped
1 teaspoon pepper
½ teaspoon cayenne pepper (optional)
1 Bay leaf
1 teaspoon Ms. Dash table blend season
3 cups chicken
8 cups organic low sodium broth
6 oz. of your choice of noodles, (I prefer egg noodles)

1 cup chopped asparagus
2 tablespoons of parsley

Directions: Heat olive oil in Dutch oven. Chop leeks and cook about 5 minutes. Add all veggies except asparagus. Add seasonings, chicken and broth. Bring to boil, add noodles reduce heat and cook until noodles are tender. Add asparagus cook 4 minutes. Add parsley and remove bay leaf before serving.

Ground Turkey Soup
1 lb. ground turkey (93% - 99% lean)
1 onion, finely chopped
6 cups vegetable broth
1 bag mixed vegetables
2 garlic cloves, finely chopped
1 can diced tomatoes
1 teaspoon red pepper flakes (optional)
1 bay leaf

Directions: Brown ground turkey, garlic and onion in a Dutch oven or a stock pot. Drain excessive fat. Add broth and bring to a boil for about 10 minutes. Add mixed vegetables, tomatoes, red pepper and bay leaf. Simmer for 20 minutes, and remove bay leaf.

Beef and Potato Soup

2 lbs. lean ground beef (bison is fine too)
2 tablespoons olive oil
4 carrots, chopped
3 celery stalks, thinly sliced
2 garlic gloves minced
1 bay leaf
2 teaspoon Worcestershire sauce
1 can organic diced tomatoes with juice
1 leek chopped
3 cups diced red potatoes
1-2 cups organic green beans (fresh or frozen)
6 cups of organic beef broth or vegetable broth
Salt and pepper to taste

Directions: Heat olive oil in Dutch oven. Add carrots, celery, garlic and leeks. Sautee for 4 minutes. Brown ground beef. Add broth, potatoes, tomatoes, seasonings and bay leaf. Cover and simmer for 30 minutes. Add remaining vegetables and cook for an additional 10 minutes. Remove bay leaf. Adjust for taste.

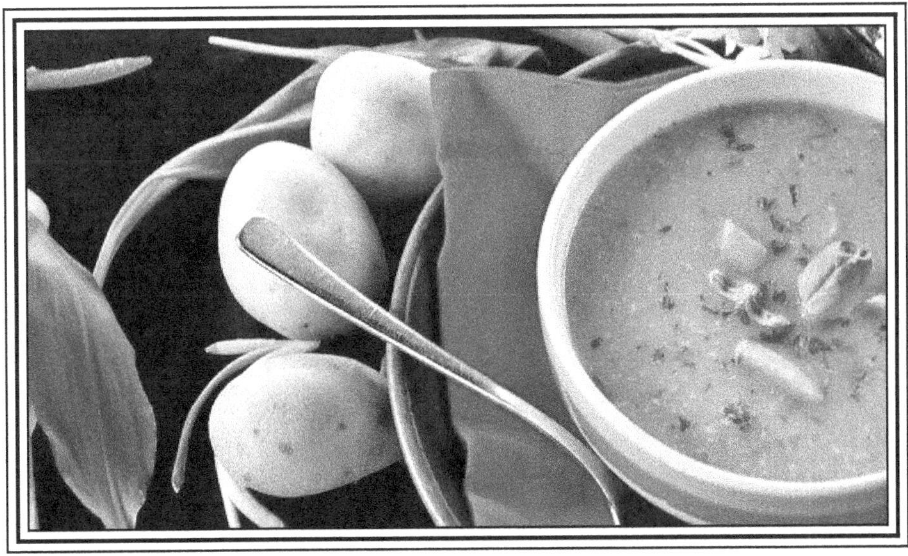

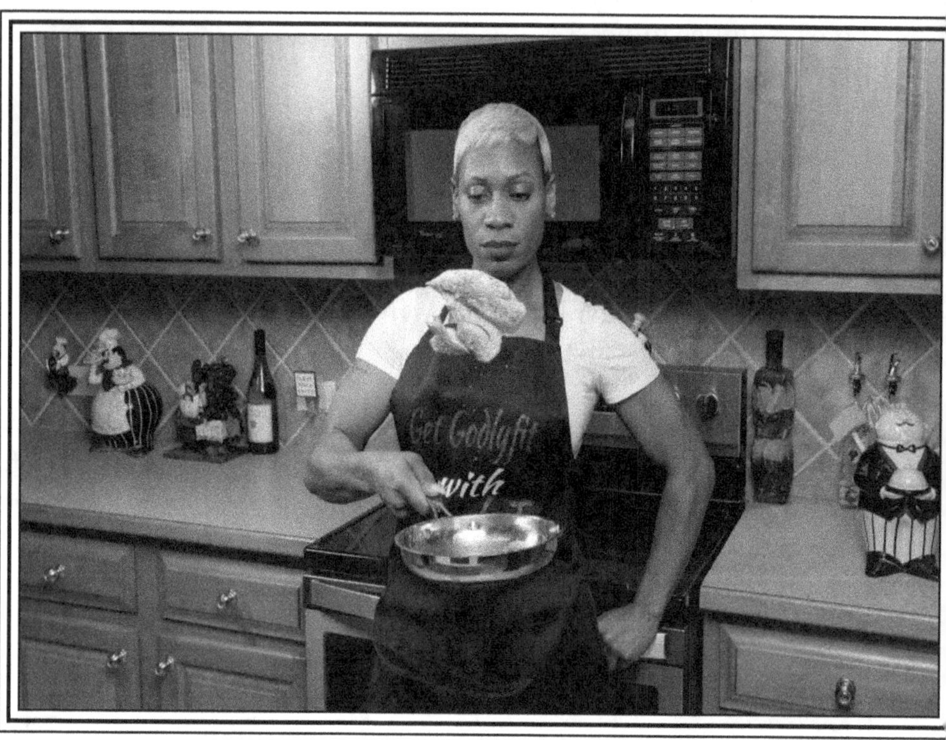
Get Godlyfit
with

<u>LUNCHES & DINNERS</u>

Grilled Chicken Breast
1 tablespoon of extra virgin olive oil
1-2 lbs. boneless chicken breast
1 ½ teaspoons sea salt
½ tsp. pepper
1 teaspoon of your favorite chicken/poultry seasoning

Directions: Wash chicken and trim excessive fat. Heat olive oil in a nonstick skillet. Make a slit on the side of the chicken; (it should look like a butterfly). Place chicken in nonstick skillet and turn over every 2 minutes. Once chicken is brown on both sides, reduce heat to almost low, then cover. Continue to turn chicken over every 4 minutes until chicken has been cooking for about 15-20 minutes. Cover to keep chicken tender and moist.

Chef Notes: Preserve the juices from chicken to use for reheating.

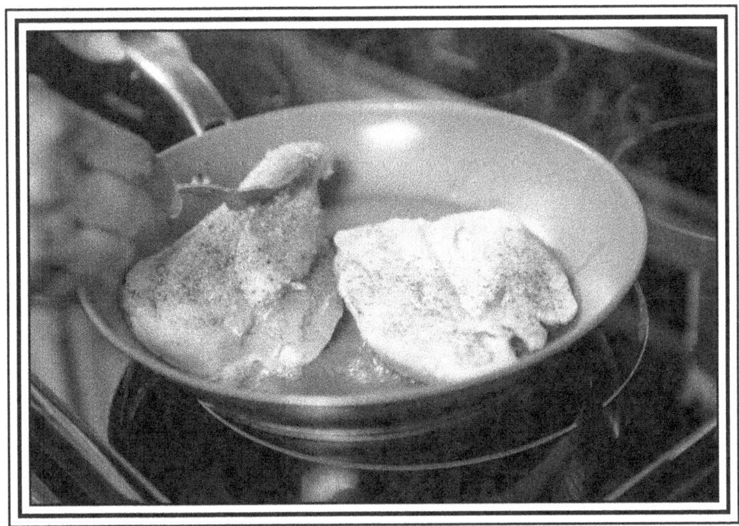

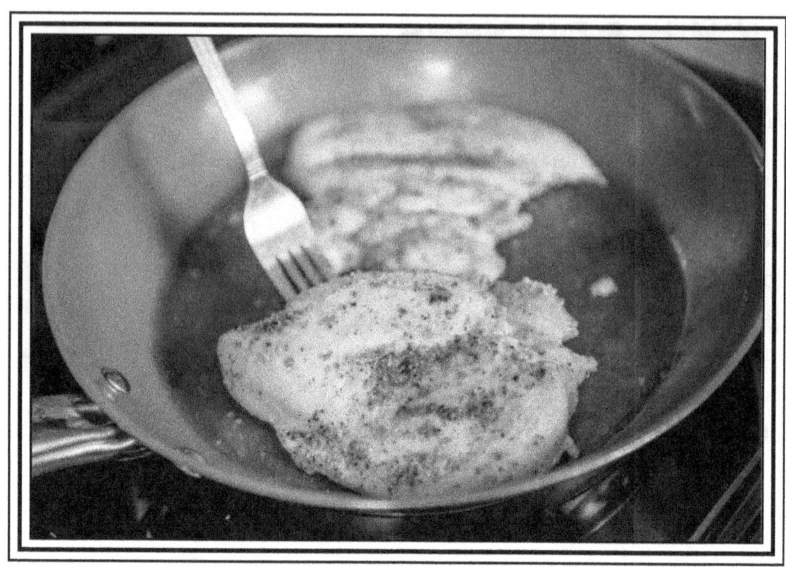

Ground Chicken Meatballs
2 tablespoons olive oil
1 lb. of 99% lean ground chicken
½ cup chopped green onion (optional)
2 tablespoons of Italian bread crumbs
Seasons of choice
1 teaspoon black pepper

Directions: Add olive oil to a skillet. Roll meatballs into 2-3 oz. ball, place apart in pan. Turn frequently to prevent sticking. Cook for 8-10 minutes. Remove from pan, place on paper towel; let sit for 2-3 minutes and serve.

Chef Notes: You may use, lean ground beef or ground turkey.

Lemon Pepper Asparagus
12-15 Asparagus spears
1 tablespoon lemon pepper seasoning (I use Ms. Dash)
1 teaspoon of salt (I use sea salt)
1 tablespoon olive oil

Directions: Place asparagus in a clean kitchen sink filled with water, to remove any errant dirt. Snip the woody end of asparagus with kitchen shears. Pre heat oven to 400 degrees. Pat dry the asparagus. Spray olive or coconut oil then drizzle your seasoning coating asparagus. Toss gentle to ensure asparagus is coated. Spread on a single layer sheet pan. Bake, roll asparagus twice. Bake 17-18 minutes. Adjust with more seasonings if desired.

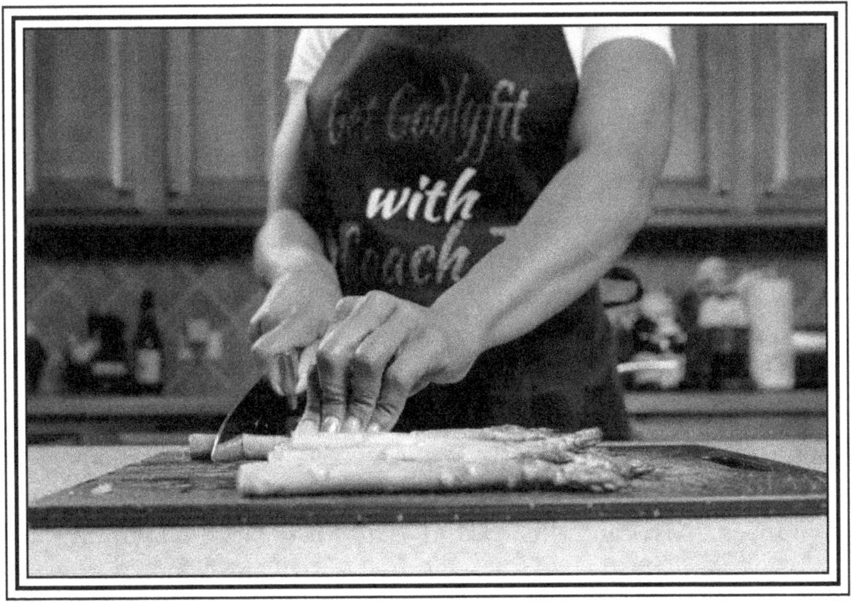

Fresh Salmon Cakes
1 tablespoon garlic and herb butter
2 tablespoons extra virgin olive oil
½ cup of onion diced
2-3 cups leftover flaked fresh salmon
1 cup of bread crumbs (I use Italian)
2 egg whites
2 tablespoons lemon juice
1 tablespoon fresh dill
1 tablespoon fresh parsley

Directions: Melt butter and cook onion until soft. Set aside. In a bowl, mix salmon, ½ cup of the bread crumbs, eggs, lemon juice, dill and parsley. Add onions and mix. Refrigerate for 20 minutes. Form into patties and dip in remaining bread crumbs. Heat skillet with olive oil and cook until golden brown. Remove from pan and top with fresh parsley.

Sweet Potato Fries
2 large sweet potatoes cut into wedges
1 ½ tablespoons extra virgin olive oil
1 tablespoon sea salt
¼ teaspoon garlic powder
¼ teaspoon smoked paprika (optional)

Directions: Preheat oven to 425 degrees. Use the top rack. In a small bowl, place potatoes and toss with olive oil and seasonings. Arrange the coated fries in a single layer on the prepared pan. Bake for 25 minutes until tender and golden. Cool for 3-5 minutes.

BROTH

2 Quarts water
1 large white onion chopped
2 carrots sliced
1 cup squash cut in cubes
1 cup rutabagas or turnips
2 celery stalks
¼ slice ginger
2 whole garlic cloves
3 stalks fresh rosemary
Sea salt to taste

Directions: Boil all ingredients for 60 minutes. Cod, strain, remove vegetable and store in container in fridge.

Chef notes: Vegetables are reusable to make more broth. Store in Mason jar for 5 days or freeze up to 3 months.

Benefits: Reduces inflammation, cleanses the liver, boost immune system, soothe digestion, contain anti-cancer properties

DETOX

Detox Bath
2 cups baking soda
2 cups Epsom salt
1-2 cups Braggs Apple Cider Vinegar
1 cup hot lemon water

Directions: Run a warm to hot bath, add all ingredients. Soak 15-20 minutes. Relax and enjoy your hot lemon water. Shower immediately to remove remaining vinegar on body.

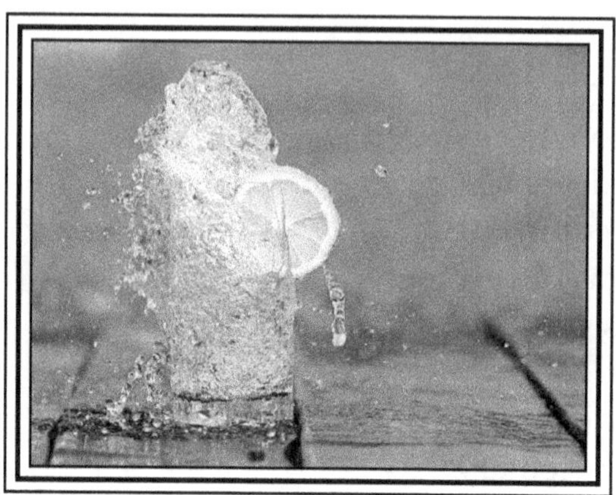

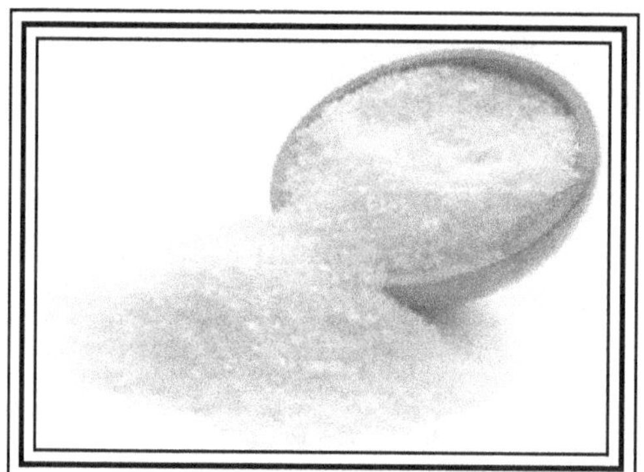

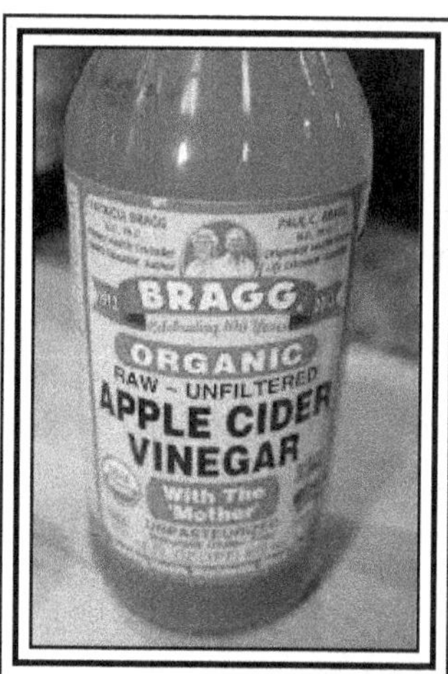

BRAGG
ORGANIC
RAW - UNFILTERED
APPLE CIDER
VINEGAR
With The
Mother

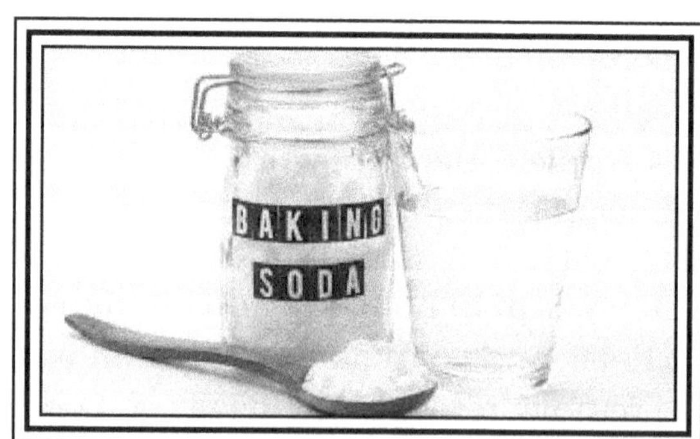

BAKING
SODA

<u>MORE BENEFITS</u>

Lemon Water
Maintain PH balance of the body
Detoxifying agent
Flushes out toxins
Help with quick weight loss
Promotes digestion
Increase metabolic rate
Helps reduce joint and muscle pain
Helps regulate natural bowel movement

Epsom Salt Bath
Reduce inflammation
Soothe muscles
Helps decrease emotional eating
Helps de-stress
Ease constipation

Braggs Vinegar
Reduces body odor
Tightens the vagina
Balances PH levels
Treat Bacteria Infection (BV)
Effective against candida

Baking Soda
Reduce inflammation
Help prevent UTI
Alkalizes the body
Prevents kidney stones

STAY CONNECTED WITH TIFFANY :

– *Bostic Total Body, LLC*
https://www.facebook.com/TiffanyBosticNC3/

- *@Godly_fitclassy*

- *Tbostic22@gmail.com*